Easy Steps to
Beauty

Easy Steps to
Beauty

A beautiful body inside and out

COSIMA GRAY

Penguin Books

Penguin Books Australia Ltd
487 Maroondah Highway, PO Box 257
Ringwood, Victoria 3134, Australia
Penguin Books Ltd
Harmondsworth, Middlesex, England
Penguin Putnam Inc.
375 Hudson Street, New York, New York 10014, USA
Penguin Books Canada Limited
10 Alcorn Avenue, Toronto, Ontario, Canada M4V 3B2
Penguin Books (NZ) Ltd
Cnr Rosedale and Airborne Roads, Albany, Auckland, New Zealand
Penguin Books (South Africa) (Pty) Ltd
5 Watkins Street, Denver Ext. 4, 2094, South Africa
Penguin Books India (P) Ltd
11, Community Centre, Panchsheel Park, New Delhi 110 017, India

First published by Penguin Books Australia Ltd 2001

3 5 7 9 10 8 6 4 2

Copyright © Penguin Books Australia Ltd 2001

Design by Marina Messiha, Penguin Design Studio
Cover image by Getty Images
Typeset in 11/16 pt Helvetica Thin by Post Pre-press Group,
Brisbane, Queensland
Printed and bound in Australia by McPherson's Printing Group, Maryborough, Victoria

National Library of Australia
Cataloguing-in-Publication data:

Gray, Cosima.
Easy steps to beauty: a beautiful body inside and out.

ISBN 0 14 100710 9.

1. Beauty, Personal. 2. Women – Health and hygiene. 3. Naturopathy. I. Title.

646.72

www.penguin.com.au

Contents

Nature gives you the face you have at twenty; it is up to you to merit the face you have at fifty.

Coco Chanel

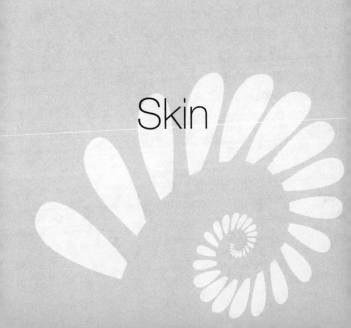

Skin

For an instant face-lift, fill a big basin or sink with cool water and put your face under water and 'bubble' for as long as your breath allows! The cold water will refresh and tighten – particularly good in summer.

Once a month dip your finger in some good olive oil and gently massage it into your face, neck and elbows. Perfect for a thorough, deep moisturise.

Choose a moisturiser that suits you.
You may alternate between a lighter
cream in summer – even a gel for
really humid days – and a heavier
cream for winter.

Wear sunscreen.
Always.

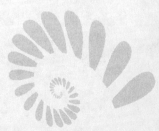

If you don't have time for a daily beauty routine, give your face a good scrub with a facecloth under the shower each morning and slap some moisturiser on (or use sunscreen instead). Use a clean facecloth again before bed at night.

Most moisturisers and skin creams
last about a year. You can tell if they
are out of date by checking the
consistency or colour. If these have
changed from when you first used
the product, then it is best
to replace them.

Youth is something very new: twenty
years ago, no one mentioned it.

Coco Chanel

Take pleasure in your beauty ritual.
Look on it as 'me' time.

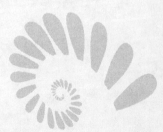

Mini-Meditation

Take five minutes to focus solely on your breath. Shut out the outside world and breathe in, breathe out. Do this first thing in the morning, in the middle of a hectic day or last thing at night.

Ideally you should cleanse, tone and moisturise twice a day. Exfoliate with a gentle scrub twice a week.

Have regular facials. Essential for the busy woman in a polluted environment.

To prevent ageing, buy a moisturiser
with a high sunscreen factor and
when outdoors wear a hat and apply
sunscreen to the face and
neck area.

Don't forget your neck – front and back! This is one area that will give away the secret of your age if you don't pamper it. Sunscreen, moisturiser and massages will help keep necks supple and creamy.

Beat blemishes by dabbing some drying mudpack on a painful pimple before bed and leaving it on overnight. This draws out all the impurities inside the volcano!

Mix your foundation with a little moisturiser to ensure a smooth complexion, particularly for a more sheer summer look. And if you do this, you won't use as much foundation.

Smile!

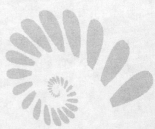

Apply blush and loose powder with the biggest brushes you can afford for a sheer, airy finish. The bigger the brush, the better. Keep your brushes clean by washing them periodically in warm soapy water and laying them horizontally to dry on a towel. If you can't afford to buy a whole kit of good brushes at once, talk to your beautician about the best range, and buy them one at a time.

Even with all my wrinkles I am beautiful!

Bessie Delaney

Your skin will need different treatments depending on the season and your age. Products that worked brilliantly last year may not now be so good for your skin. You can always ask someone at a cosmetics counter for advice on the most suitable product for you – even if you don't buy their expensive version of it.

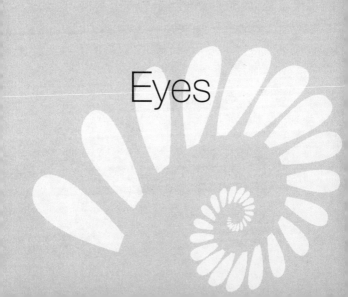

Eyes

Buy some good sunglasses with proper UV protection. Use them in harsh light.

Dab a tiny amount of eye gel around the eyes, particularly underneath, as soon as you get out of the shower in the morning. Wait a little while before moisturising, then apply concealer if it was a particularly big night.

A girl's best friend – so say many models – is the eyelash curler. Invest in a good one – metal, not plastic – and use it to crimp the lashes before applying mascara or eyeshadow. This 'opens up' the eyes and dramatically enhances the effect of mascara and eye make-up.

For dark and luscious lashes, use a lash-extending mascara. There are plenty available now in all price ranges.

Eyeshadow is best applied with a small brush rather than the padded applicator supplied. A brush gives a sheer look and a better application of colour, and avoids a 'drawn on' look.

The key to a good, clump-free mascara is the brush, so check out the brushes supplied with mascaras before you buy. A further tip to avoid clumping is to hold the brush loosely in tissue or a piece of toilet paper for a few seconds before applying. Some people recommend waving the wand in the air to allow the mascara to set slightly before applying.

If you don't like a made-up look,
or are sensitive to eye make-up,
consider getting your lashes tinted.
Most beauticians use mild vegetable
dyes that will keep your lashes dark
and glossy for six to eight weeks.

Eyebrows frame the face. Keep them shapely with a professional wax once in a while, and use tweezers between times to maintain the shape. Pay attention to stray hairs between and underneath the brows, but where possible don't pluck from 'above' the eyebrow, as this interferes with the natural line.

Contrary to popular opinion, eyes are not always enhanced by dark liner or shadow. If you're worried about looking tired, the best method is to use an eyelash curler as outlined on page 24, and then apply a matte light or cream coloured shadow on the lids. This brightens the eyes.

Place moistened chamomile teabags
on closed eyelids for ten minutes to
revive tired, strained and puffy eyes.

'I want to grow old without facelifts . . . I want to have the courage to be loyal to the face I have made.'

Marilyn Monroe

The best-kept secret: a brow pencil. Use light, quick strokes of a freshly sharpened brow pencil, slightly darker than your brow colour, to define the shape.

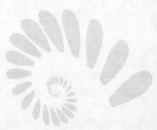

To revive tired-looking eyes, use a pale, shimmery colour of eyeshadow. Sweep the shadow under your brows to open up the eye area, then use a small brush to dab the same shimmer on the inner corners of your eyes to banish dark shadows.

What you can't live without
Mascara
Soft brush
Gentle eye make-up remover
Eye gel
Concealer

Lips

Dry lips? This may sound painful, but gently exfoliating winter lips with an old soft toothbrush works wonders. Apply vaseline or lip balm afterwards.

Lip liner adds definition to lips. Choose one that matches your lips exactly or is a shade darker. Fill in with a lighter-coloured lipstick to give you pretty, pouting lips. For extra pout, dab with gloss.

For berry lips and cherub cheeks,
use a rose-pink lipstick. Swipe
lipstick straight from the tube onto
lips, then finger-dab colour onto
cheeks, blending towards the hairline
before the colour sets.

If you find a lipstick you really love,
go back and buy four more. It may
be discontinued next season.

What you can't live without
Red lipstick

41

Five Essential Handbag Items

sunscreen
handcream
lip gloss
small bottle of fragrance
nail file

Teeth

Keep a toothbrush and toothpaste
in a little cosmetics bag at work.
Yes, brushing your teeth in the loos
is daggy, but not as daggy as
going for a filling!

Floss your teeth every day – even between the teeth right at the back – to prevent gum disease and to keep your breath fresh.

Use a whitening toothpaste to brush morning and night, and before you go out.

Mini-Meditation

Lie comfortably on the floor. As you breathe in, imagine that the breath is golden light. Visualise the light touching every cell in your body. Breathe out. Repeat four or five times. This meditation is very healing.

If you use mouthwash for fresh breath, avoid those containing alcohol. They tend to dry out the mouth and worsen the problem.

Have an annual check-up at the dentist. In this case, prevention is certainly better than the cure!

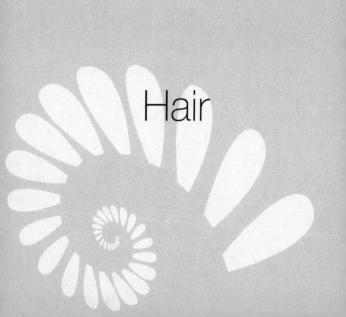

Hair

Keep your hairbrush clean by combing out loose hair and washing the brush in warm water with a tiny bit of shampoo. A clean brush means clean hair.

If you've always wondered how you
would look with short hair or a
radically different style, be brave!
Book yourself into a super salon
and do it.

To keep locks healthy, get a trim
every six to eight weeks and while
you're there, have the roots redone.

If you have dry or coloured hair, give it a good deep-conditioning treatment once a month.

Quick fix for oily hair: blondes can comb through some talcum powder to get rid of the oily look if you don't have time to wash it!

No matter what type of hair you have, opt for styling products that contain shine-enhancing ingredients, such as silicone, or light-reflecting botanicals.

What you can't live without

Diamante or floral hair clips

Good-quality shampoo

and conditioner

The shine factor!

Hands and Feet

Take a footbath each week.
Pour warm water into a basin and
add a sprinkle of bath salts or a few
drops of your favourite essential oil.
Let your tired feet soak for fifteen
minutes or so, then pat dry and
apply foot lotion. It won't change your
life, but you'll feel pampered.

Always use gloves when gardening, washing the dishes and cleaning.

Rub tired feet with peppermint lotion
or a dash of peppermint essential oil.

Reflexology is a holistic therapy in which it is believed that the various parts of the foot correspond to parts of the body. Massaging certain reflex points on the feet unblocks energy and helps the body heal itself. You will feel invigorated.

Exfoliate hands with a gentle scrub
once a week. Great for keeping
them smooth.

Use sunscreen on your hands or
wear gloves when driving in the sun.

For dry hands, apply a good dollop of handcream just before you go to bed. The next day your hands will be silky smooth.

Mini-Meditation

Breathe in. State one thing you want to achieve this week. Breathe out. Tell yourself how you will achieve it. Breathe in and repeat what you want to achieve. Breathe out. How will you achieve it? Know that it will happen.

Sprinkle the contents of three green-tea bags into a large bowl of warm water. Soak your feet for fifteen minutes, then use a foot-buffing scrub and a pumice stone to smooth stubborn calluses.

Keep a handcare pamper pack
handy – at work or in your handbag –
that contains essentials like nail files,
clippers, handcream and a clear or
light-coloured polish.

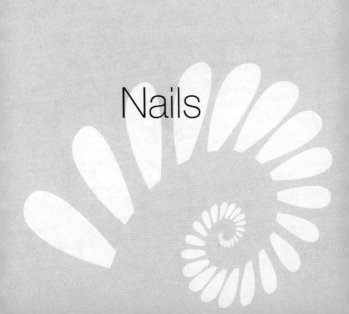

Nails

A very pale pinky-purple polish on fingernails will make you look more tanned, even if your skin has just a bit of golden colour. Try it.

Almond or apricot kernel oils are great for massaging into cuticles. Push back your half-moons gently with a fingernail after you've had a shower, when the skin is soft.

Paint fingernails without painting the cuticles – get someone else to do it!

If you are shy about letting your toenails see the light of day, remove dry skin from around the cuticles of the toes after a long soak, then trim your nails and paint them. Lilac, burgundy, silver – explore and have fun.

Don't chew your fingernails or the
skin around them.

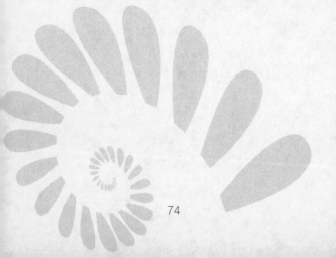

Put cottonwool balls in between your toes when painting your toenails.

Brittle nails can mean you are suffering from a deficiency in iron or zinc. Natural supplements can improve the nails.

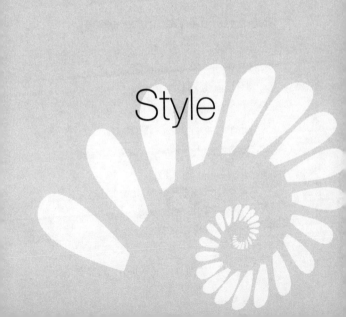

Style

Five Essential Wardrobe Items

knee-length black dress
fitted jumper
crisp white shirt
bright or patterned scarf
well-tailored winter coat

Wear simple black or a dark-coloured suit or dress rather than two colours for the most flattering effect. Two colours tend to cut you in half. Save the splash of colour for the scarf and accessories.

Get your colours done by a specialist. Based on skin tones, hair and eye colour, this analysis will give you a palette of ideal colours to wear for someone with your looks. Throw out everything in your wardrobe that is taboo, and discover colours that you thought you could never wear.

Cotton undies are best.

Always keep a spare pair of stockings in the cupboard and your desk drawer. Ladders will occur at the most inopportune moments.

Accessorise sensibly. Wear just one
or two striking pieces.

If you have a pale complexion and blonde hair, you are probably a **Water** element. With your blue–green eyes and rosy cheeks, you feel most comfortable in soft, layered garments. Yellow-based reds and browns are not for you.

Fire women look fab in dramatic shades – burgundy, hot pink and orange – all at once, if you dare. Discreet colours don't do you justice. How do you know if fire is your element? Your locks are rich and dark and your skin has subtle yellow undertones.

Delicate and fair **Air** women – with
your reddish or honey-blonde mane,
you're always a whirlwind of activity.
Elegant and understated in dress,
you look best in pastels and neutrals,
but don't be dragged down by dark
or dull colours.

Earth women glow in the colours of autumn, from golden yellows to pine-green hues. Highlight your eyes with burnt orange and put some sparkle on your lips. Browny reds do best justice to your olive skin and chestnut tresses.

If you're not keen on scaling the heights and wearing high heels, then kitten-style mules and slides are the answer. With a finely sculpted heel, these shoes are low enough to keep you grounded while still being the epitome of elegance.

It's amazing how good-quality,
matching bra and knickers will make
you feel. Invest and enjoy.

Are you a true fashionista? This doesn't have to be an expensive habit. Maintain a wardrobe of key classics such as tailored trousers or a well-cut suit, then buy one or two funky pieces each season, such as a diamante belt, a frilly flamenco top or a clutch in a bright colour.

Healthy
Woman
Food

Begin each day with a hot drink
made from the juice of one lemon
and boiling water to cleanse the liver
and kick-start your metabolism.
It's also an excellent source of
vitamin C. Add some finely chopped
ginger for extra zing.

Try a filling banana smoothie as a healthy breakfast or lunch substitute. Use soy milk occasionally and don't forget a dash of honey, a couple of spoonfuls of yoghurt and a teaspoon of wheat hearts. Mmm. Add a few strawberries for an even better taste.

Don't be alarmed by the thought of detoxing. It's not about eating nothing but watermelon for four weeks. Instead, try to have one or two days each month when you eat only fresh, organic food.

Drink one or two glasses of alcohol each week as a special treat, rather than out of habit every night. Alcohol dehydrates your body and starves it of essential vitamins.

Mini-Meditation

Imagine a wave. You are riding the crest of the wave. Your body is gently caressed by the water. You are carried along effortlessly. Breathe. You can smell the salt water.

Smoking is so passé. It stains teeth,
makes clothes smell and will, in time,
create lines around your mouth
and eyes.

Carbohydrates are essential for every woman's good health. They ensure excellent concentration and longer-lasting energy. Make sure you eat enough pasta, brown rice and bread – approximately four serves per day.

Flush out toxins each morning
with this vinegar drink. Add
1 teaspoon (or more if you prefer) of
apple cider vinegar and a heaped
teaspoon of honey to a cup of boiling
water. Drink it down and feel revived.

If you are not feeling on top of things, your body may need some nutritional supplements such as vitamin B or iron. Discuss this with your doctor or naturopath.

Indulge in health drinks such as
carrot, apple and orange juice.
The essential vitamins and minerals
go straight into the blood stream.
Make sure you drink them on an
empty stomach for best effects.

Try to eat seasonally. Buy nectarines and stone fruit in summer; pears, figs and pumpkins in autumn; oranges and mandarins in winter; and asparagus in spring. In season, fruit and vegetables are full of natural flavour.

Drink green tea – it is full of antioxidants.

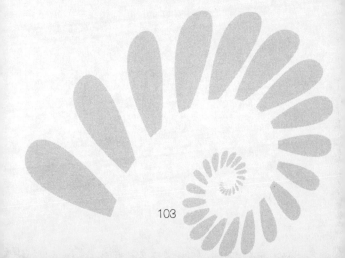

Eat plenty of fresh vegetables, especially green leafy ones, which are full of iron.

Stale breath can be banished by chewing fresh parsley – stalks and all! Keep a pot on your windowsill and munch away after dinner.

Mini-Meditation

Take five minutes to concentrate briefly on every part of your body. Consciously acknowledge your toes, your elbows and your ears. Be aware of how your body feels physically.

Drink water. We all know this, but why is it so important? Water can play an important part in relieving backache, lethargy, headaches and constipation.

Feeling tired? Next time you feel lilke a caffeine hit, try fresh juice instead. It will revitalise you, won't stress your system and, after a few weeks without caffeine, you will see your skin start to glow. Try juicing beetroot with some apple and ginger. It sounds awful, looks glorious and tastes too good to be true.

In moments of weakness, choose
dark chocolate over milk chocolate –
dark chocolate is an antioxidant.

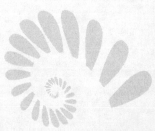

Eliminate tea and coffee from
your diet for a couple of days
each month.

I swear by hot Ribena. A cup of this after an exhausting moment is very restorative.

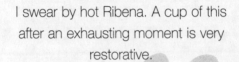

Bodily Bliss

Yoga and Pilates are excellent for balanced bodies and minds. They are particularly good for fragile backs.

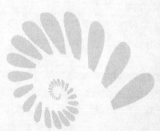

The best thing you can add to a bath is oats. Cut the foot off an old (clean) stocking and fill it with natural oats. Tie a knot in the top and throw it in the water or hang it under the running tap. It makes the bath milky and naturally moisturises your skin.

Ideally, we should all be exercising for about an hour each day. If you just don't have time, then try to walk whenever possible – to the corner shop, to the train station, with the dog. Walking is the best exercise for fat loss and for keeping your metabolism active.

Take five slow, deep breaths every
hour to reoxygenate and energise
your body and calm your mind.

Good sex – often.

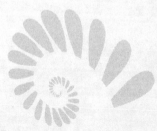

Self-examine your breasts once
a month, checking for any lumps
or bumps.

Sit up straight at your desk
or when driving.

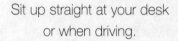

Add essential oils to your bath:
ylang ylang for soothing, geranium
for balancing, clary sage for
hormonal moments (but do not use
this during pregnancy).

Exercise every day for a healthier
body and a better night's sleep.

A brisk walk every day keeps you
trim and the blood flowing.

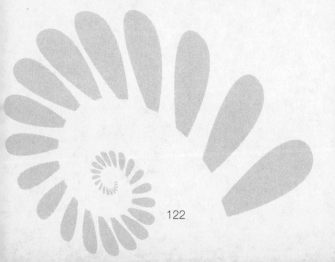

A few drops of echinacea at the
first sign of a cold or flu can
work wonders.

Sleep.

Mini-Meditation

*Think about how you want to feel . . .
independent, filled with wonder,
healthy, vital, balanced, loved, open,
secure, strong. Write down these
thoughts. Work out how you will
achieve them: 'Do yoga once a
week', 'Be childlike from time to
time', 'Get close to nature' or
'Nurture myself with a pedicure'.
At the end of the week, look at how
you have progressed.*

Sit under a shady tree. Soak up the good energy and let your muscles release all their tension.

Go for a walk along the beach and soak up those negative ions, or walk in the bush and smell the fresh air. There is nothing like cleansing the body with a lungful of fresh air.

Wear a proper sports bra accredited by the AIS when exercising, to prevent breasts sagging.

Include some stretches in your busy day. Do five minutes of gentle stretching after your shower each morning to feel limbered up and invigorated.

For the ultimate in pampering, book into a spa or retreat for an hour – or a day, if you can afford it. Have a facial, a massage and a reflexology treatment.

Go for a swim in the ocean as often as possible. The ocean water invigorates the body and can make you feel thoroughly cleansed.

Don't forget to loofah in between waxes to prevent in-grown hairs.

Travel Tips

Travel in style. Wear comfortable clothes on the plane. Layers work particularly well. Keep a smart neckscarf with you for when you arrive.

Dab on a little eye gel
every six hours when flying.

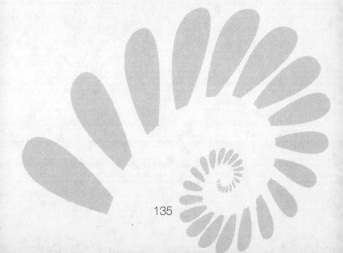

Mini-Meditation

Imagine you are in a rainforest. There is sunlight warming your back. You can hear birds calling. A leaf falls gently from a high tree. Breathe. You are at peace.

Drink lots of water before and during a long flight. Keep an Evian spray handy and rehydrate your face often. Brush your hair and put on some lipstick before leaving the plane.

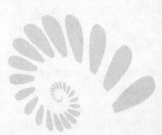

Keep a small bottle of fragrance or
deodorant handy on long flights
or car trips.

If you do a lot of air travel, wiggle your ankles and wrists vigorously every hour. Massage your calves and walk up and down the aisle.

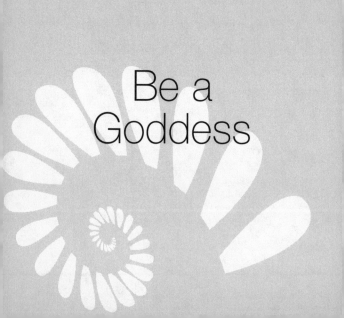

Be a
Goddess

Take up belly dancing. Curves are
natural and sexy.

In the few days before your period, be extra kind to yourself. Have some early nights and quiet time, drink lots of water and reduce your caffeine intake. Make allowances for mood swings or feelings of irritation and anger.

Look at how your parents have aged.
Genetics play a strong role in how
we look and feel as the years go by.
What can you do to improve on this
inheritance? Stop smoking, release
long-held resentment or take a little
more time for 'you'? Make it happen.

Get eight hours of sleep each night.
Night-time is when the body goes
into action and your cells are
renewed and replenished. Eight
hours' sleep will also help keep the
panda eyes under control.

If you want the 'I've just been to Noosa' look, apply fake tan and go over it with a light dusting of bronze powder. Your friends will never know the difference.

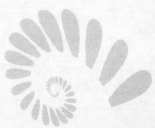

Face your demons. What has happened in your life that you haven't yet dealt with? You may feel fine, but deep down you may need to resolve issues that will rise up and take their toll later in life. It requires courage and honesty, and you may need some help, but ultimately you will be liberated.

Love your body.

Cultivate inner calm and serenity.
Build a little wall around yourself to
block out negative people. Don't take
other people's problems on board –
listen and help, but don't let them
pull you down too.

The most beautiful people are those
who radiate happiness. This means
that the secret to beauty lies in doing
what feels right for you and being
good to people, including yourself.

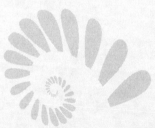

In the words of Bridget Jones:
'inner poise'.

Be sure to nurture your creativity.
You may not be a gifted artist, but
using paints, coloured pencils or
words to express what you feel will
tap into an inner creativity. Make time
to do this.

You can take no credit for beauty at sixteen. But if you are beautiful at sixty, it will be your soul's own doing.

Marie Stopes

Cosima Gray has just discovered
the joys of good handcream
and twinsets.

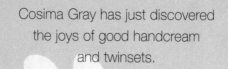